PROGESTERONE:

The Ultimate Woman's Feel Good Hormone

By Dan Purser MD

www.drpurser.com

D1245400

ACKNOWLEDGEMENTS

I just would be totally remiss if I did not start off by thanking a master educator, Neal Rouzier, MD of the Clinics of the Palm Deserts – he has introduced so many physicians to a "wiser" practice of preventive medicine through the modern medical literature. So many of us would have been lost (and still would be) without him wandering still in the desert of medical misinformation. And thanks to one of the kindest, nicest, and smartest physicians on the planet – Michael Jensen, MD – my best friend and one of the most awesome football players I know.

And to the team at MedQuest Pharmacy in Bountiful, Utah – the best compounding pharmacy team on the planet. Thanks for the years of great education!

And for Nayan Patel, PhD at Central Drug in La Habra, California and USC – thanks for the golden nuggets and for making one of the best progesterones on the planet.

And thanks to my wonderful wife and her daughters – the info I've gained from watching how you use the progesterone is invaluable – and thanks for the loving support – I love you Denise and your womanly behaviors and needs!

-Dan Purser, MD

Your Free Bonus

As a Small Token of Thanks for buying this book, I'd like to offer a FREE Bonus Gift EXCLUSIVE to my readers.

You can download my **PURSER Preferred Lab Solutions PDF** contains 10+ pages of very valuable and crucial info you'll need to move forward.

In this FREE Bonus you'll learn:

-- Labs you should get if you wish to know where your pituitary and hormone levels are falling.

-- What proper ranges should be! (Not what some lab director thinks they might be...)

-- The list of labs needed for a Complete Female Panel or Complete Male Panel

-- Downloadable and Printable so you can give it to your doctor

-- Directions for you to go to my website to access Direct Labs™ to order and pay for yourself when no one else will help you.

You can download the free gift here (**PLUS other REALLY VALUABLE BONUSES**):

www.drpurser.com

It's SUPER EASY!

My Legal Protection

Progesterone: The Ultimate Women's Feel Good Hormone

© 2014 DAN PURSER MD

loss of health or other medical issues that arise from the material represented herein.

Do not use the information contained in this book to treat yourself. Please consult with a knowledgeable physician in your area before starting any treatment as possibly suggested in this book. I will not be held responsible if something goes wrong. So BE CAREFUL! Thank you.

FOREWORD

By Keith Radley

I've known and been close friends with Dr. Dan Purser for 12 years now, and even gave him key ideas and direction for his/our textbook **PROGRAM 120: A Physician's Handbook on ProActive Preventive Medicine.** I also watched him slowly recover from a hideous wreck that almost cost him is life – it was a long and arduous recovery, one that most people did not think he could come back from – yes, his is one of *those* stories. In the end his recovery was amazing! And now, looking back, this is a man who has done it all – survived trauma of all sorts – legal, physical, mental, and love disasters -- for more than a year and a half he could not even walk or talk – and now he lectures all over the world about preventive medicine issues for women and men. It's amazing – he actually relishes going in front of and speaking to big groups – 5000 people or more – showing anyone who's interested, including hundreds of physicians, how to proactively deal with prevention issues in a hugely beneficial way, and in the process saving thousands of lives.

He practices what he preaches. He's felt your pain – maybe worse. He knows what most patients have gone through because he's gone through it himself.

What more needs to be said?

INTRODUCTION

I work in a plastic surgery group where I often deal with healing problems (to clarify –caused by problems from outside our office) on patients where wounds won't heal correctly plus I've written a textbook for physicians on proactive preventive care that's gotten a lot of interest. Through a number of odd and life-saving events I also am lucky enough to perform pituitary endocrinology research in Los Angeles with arguably the best pituitary endocrinologist in the world, Nabil Gemayel, MD (who's also a cardiologist and is on staff at the University of Southern California). I and my wife have decided I must do this research for penitence for past sins (I'm pretty sure) because there's no reimbursement for travel or time – it's volunteer -- we're just trying to help people and figure out very complex disease processes. Through this work, and my office, I repeatedly see a lot of women who are suffering with migraines, hot flashes, night sweats and PMS. I think it's amazing that these female patients find me who have the most horrific problems. And the one hormone I almost always prescribe to these women is the ultimate feel good hormone – progesterone.

Progesterone gets rid of hot flashes, night sweats, migraines, PMS, and more. It is wonderful. And highly under-appreciated by my fellow physicians and most patients,

I'm talking about compounded human progesterone (usually called P4 in studies) – and I mostly use a sublingual triturate (though I've developed some awesome topical progesterone products for various companies). Let me say up front, for those of you who've tried it, and thought it didn't work very well if at all, that the quality of the progesterone makes a huge difference – a difference between not working and changing your life back to normal. Or you were scared away by a well-meaning but unknowledgeable doctor who said bad things about it – well, I speak all around the country about preventive medicine issues – mostly to physicians and occasionally to (very large) crowds of regular women who are suffering, and human progesterone (P4) is just about completely harmless (we'll get in to this more later) and almost totally beneficial.

If it was not safe, why else would women who are pregnant make so much of it when they were carrying that tiny basically unprotected human life?

Exactly – let's look at the studies and the research.

Chapter 1

What is "NATURAL" Progesterone?

Progesterone (4-pregnene-3, 20-dione or P4 in this case[1]) is the "feel good" hormone of pregnancy. We are strictly talking about naturally occurring biologically identical human progesterone – not synthetic progestational agents such as progestin, medroxyprogesterone acetate, or norethisterone – these are not the natural progesterone and are very problematic and side effect intensive (they have almost exactly the opposite side effects when compared to the benefits of natural progesterone).

Known Side Effects From Taking Medroxyprogesterone (Provera® or MPA)

(Studies are legion, look at Pub Med for more supporting articles)

MPA is a teratogen and cannot be used in pregnancy[2].
MPA increases cholesterol and increases risk of heart disease[3].
MPA increases foam cell formation, endothelial inflammation, plaque formation, strokes and heart attacks[4].
MPA is carcinogenic and causes breast cancer[5] (see PEPI[6] trial).
MPA has no effect on osteoporosis (i.e. does not help)[7].
MPA is associated with side effects of increased bleeding, bloating, and depression[8].

MPA provides a serum progesterone level of zero – it is immeasurable as progesterone.

Why? MPA IS NOT PROGESTERONE[9]!

What does all of this mean? Synthetic progestins are *not* safe – period. The literature is clear on this whether used in a birth control pill or otherwise, THEY ARE NOT SAFE. We rarely, if ever, will give them on our practice.

Chapter 2

Levels

This may be a new concept for you but, yes, you can and should get serum progesterone levels -- monthly until they are at a therapeutic level (> 10 ng/ml – 20 ng/ml) then at least annually thereafter.

"Normal" P4 Values[10]

- Female (pre-ovulation): less than 1 ng/mL
- Female (mid-cycle): 5 to 20 ng/mL
- Male: less than 1 ng/mL
- Postmenopausal: less than 1 ng/mL
- 1st trimester: 11.2-90.0 ng/mL
- 2nd trimester: 25.6-89.4 ng/mL
- 3rd trimester: 48.4-42.5 ng/mL

Initial Levels

On initial exam most patients will have near zero progesterone levels if they are menopausal. They may be taking some OTC natural progesterone product which might give them a little in their serum (but this would require a LOT of natural OTC progesterone). *[They could bathe in a natural progesterone cream 24 hours a day and not get therapeutic levels – Program 120 Ed.]*

Ideal Levels

You want progesterone levels to be 10 ng/mL or greater (up to but not above 20 ng/ml) for optimal protection from breast[11] and uterine cancer. We disagree with Hargrove in not regularly checking levels as our experience has shown that if levels are too high for a long time you can get significant weight gain and maximal acinar and minimal ductal and stromal cell proliferation of the breast and vagina[12].

Problem Levels

There are no levels that are too high because in pregnancy you can see levels that are in the 200-400 ng/ml range. But for the above reasons keep them below 30 ng/ml.

If levels climb above 50 or 100 ng/ml? **Look for pregnancy!**

Chapter 3

50+ Researched Benefits (and Warnings) of Biologically Identical Human Progesterone (P4)

Natural progesterone (P4), when levels are optimized (>10 ng/ml), effectively, gives the following AMAZING benefits (this is why I've written a #1 Amazon bestseller (in Health) and done a whole UDEMY course on this incredibly important hormone and how women can and should get it for personal use.) *(FYI: RDT = Rapid Dissolve Triturate):*

1. Natural progesterone lowers cholesterol *[at 200 mgm of micronized progesterone a day in one PEPI study arm[13]]*(Especially when given in conjunction with E2)[14].
2. Natural progesterone (P4) elevates HDL levels (hard to do)[15].
3. Decreases foam cell formation[16], endothelial inflammation, plaque formation, and thus strokes and risk of heart attacks[17].
4. Decreases breast density and thus breast cancer[18].
5. Decreases breast cancer risk by 5.4X (540%) when levels are "normal" (>10 ng/ml)[19].
6. Decreases risk of death from ALL cancers 10X
7. when levels are normal (>10 ng/ml)[20].
8. Natural progesterone cause apoptosis ("pops") almost all breast cancer cells[21] PLUS reduces breast cancer causing genes by 75%[22] – that's why it is allowed be to sold OTC

(in tiny amounts) by the FDA (so when your doctor says it causes cancer and he looks all stunned you want it just laugh and tell him that).

9. Increases bone density preventing osteoporosis and related fractures[23].

10. Prevents and treats endometrial hyperplasia (use triple or quadruple the usual dose)[24].

11. If you give enough, progesterone almost always halts uterine bleeding (cyclical bleeding)[25]. A HUGE benefit if you have benign menorrhagia or metrorrhagia.

12. Can act as a hypersomniac (sleep aid) if you give 100-200 mgm at night orally for sleep[26] problems. Orally administered progesterone may have advantages over other routes of administration in the treatment of premenstrual syndrome (PMS) because of substantially higher levels of the anxiolytic metabolites 5 alpha and 5 beta pregnenolone[27] which also cause drowsiness[28].

13. Oral P4 also treats peri-menopausal symptoms (also called PMS) in the same manner (give double or triple the usual dose for about a week)[29].

14. Oral (and some topical) P4 will also get rid of 98% of hot flushes (flashes) and night sweats in pre and post-menopausal women[30].

15. A study at UCLA showed natural progesterone reduces endothelial inflammation reducing the risk of stroke and heart attack (MI)[31].

16. Remember – natural oral micronized progesterone (given sublingually as a troche and/or RDT) has improved bioavailability and much fewer reported side effects compared with synthetic progestins[32].

17. P4, when given with estradiol, improves the quality of life according to a Mayo Clinic report[33]. (NONE of my patients would EVER argue with this statement.)

18. Improves libido (along with testosterone)[34].

19. WARNING: Synthetic progestins (i.e. medroxyprogesterone acetate, norgesterol, etc), on the

other hand, often cause androgenic side effects (acne, body and facial hair), depression, and weight gain. Natural micronized progesterone is devoid of the androgenic effects on the lipid profile seen with MPA and other synthetic progestational agents; for that reason, it may be preferable in HRT protocols for peri-menopausal and postmenopausal women[35].

20. When given the choice, women in Australia much preferred more natural compounded (though difficult to find) progesterone than synthetics[36]. (This same is true around the world for ALL women.)

21. Progesterone causes a direct increase in BMD (bone mineral density) in women with osteoporosis or osteopenia[37].

22. Progesterone can increase libido in women and helps with HSDD (Hypoactive Sexual Desire Disorder)[38].

23. Progesterone causes an improvement in insulin receptor function (prevents diabetes)[39].

24. Progesterone causes weight loss or normalization in most studies (NOT gain)[40].

25. Men should not take progesterone unless they are a sex offender in jail[41] (it decreases libido).

26. Normal premenopausal progesterone levels (in women) are 4-25 ng/ml. Optimal levels are a little tighter at 10-20 ng/ml.

27. Only get serum progesterone levels not salivary or urinary levels[42] (because they are completely inaccurate). This salivary approach, though highly touted on the internet, is not supported in the literature as being accurate.

28. Usually biologically identical human progesterone is given (and preferred by patients[43]) as a flavored triturate or troche under the tongue until it dissolves (no chewing or swallowing if they can help it and do not drink or eat ten minutes before or after taking) -- topically expect poor absorption (except through mucosal membrane)[44] [45].

29. Expect dizziness with a high dose[46] so take right before bed.

30. Expect nipple tenderness (but it's rare) – back off the dose if that's the case.
31. Natural progesterone acts like a natural anxiolytic/sedative/hypnotic – good, but if a patient has this effect with their progesterone then do not take in the AM[47].
32. Oral (swallowed as in a capsule) progesterone undergoes first pass effects in liver – sublingual triturate (RDT) does not[48] so it's not wasted in the liver.
33. Again men should not use – progesterone severely inflames vascular endothelium[49] and causes impotence!
34. Female postmenopausal patient with insomnia? Change her progesterone to a capsule form and give the 100-400 mgm as Prometrium® or compounded progesterone capsules (neither my first preference) orally at night. (Helps her stop the addicting sleep medications.)
35. Natural progesterone helps with stress and acts as a natural anxiolytic AND protects the nerves from damage[50].
36. Natural progesterone is very mood[51] elevating especially the next morning after you take it.
37. That numbness and tingling in your fingertips? That gut/digestive problem? (You thought it was IBS.) Those weird heart palpitations that come and go? (HAH! I got you now because NO DOCTOR has ever asked you about those, right? Bet you've kept those a secret…). Those could all be from demyelination of either the Vagal Nerve or the peripheral nerves. Lack of adequate progesterone production can cause failure of the myelin and glia[52] – the protective covering around the nerves. Adequate progesterone levels helps myelin recover[53] and return (yes, even somewhat in MS[54])(and in diabetic neuropathy[55]).
38. Along with #36, according to the prestigious journal NEUROTRAUMA -- natural progesterone is VERY neuroprotecting and can help women (not men) recover from traumatic brain injury and heal their brain[56].
39. Remember Hargrove, JT et al from *Infertility and Reproductive Clinics of North America*[57] *(he was the chair*

of the Menopause Clinic at Vanderbilt University Medical Center):

1. Titrate progesterone to pre-menopausal levels. Give 1, 2, 3, or 4 100 mgm progesterone a day to achieve this if you need to – don't be shy. Progesterone is protective!

2. Treat menopause as deficiency state.

3. Correct all hormone levels that are deficient (remember: it's the hormonal milieu!).

4. Use human micronized bio-identical hormones[58].

5. Metabolized by normal metabolic pathways.

6. This approach avoids problem causing metabolites.

7. There is absolutely NO reason to not give progesterone to ALL postmenopausal women – hysterectomy or not.

8. There is no good reason NOT to give these bio-identical estrogens and progesterone every day[59]. *Do not cycle – give them all every day.*

40. WARNING: PREGNANCY PROBLEM: You have a patient on HRT and her level of progesterone comes back >100 ng/ml, why? She's pregnant until proven otherwise.

41. Some women, with bad endometriosis (usually terrible endometriosis) desire to take a LOT of progesterone – and this is alright – let them because they probably have "progesterone resistance" (progesterone endometrial receptor dysfunction or absence[60]) and feel better (for probably the first time in their lives) when taking lots of sublingual progesterone RDTs. This occurs in about 1 out of 100 (1-2%) of women with endometriosis. They will have NO side effects (drowsiness etc) from taking the 14-17 progesterone RDTs at night (!!??!) and running really high serum progesterone levels but it will save their lives, marriages, careers and brains.

42. PMS PROBLEM: You have a pre-menopausal patient with bad PMS symptoms, what can you do? Use P4 in a 100 mgm compounded vaginal suppository for 7-14 days (prior and up to menstruation).

43. POST-PARTUM BLUES PROBLEM: You have a patient with bad post-partum depression, what can you do? Start on 100 mgm TID sublingual P4 for 7 days, then twice per day

sublingual P4 for 7 days, then daily (sublingually) P4 for 7 days[61].

44. HOT FLASH PROBLEM: You have a perimenopausal patient with bad hot flashes (Inhibin A in decline from the ovary is *now* felt to cause hot flashes), night sweats, and vaginal dryness -- what can you do? Start on 100 mgm TID sublingual (RDT) P4 for 7 days (or until symptoms resolve) realizing they won't cycle (but who cares? Right?).

45. MIGRAINE PROBLEM: You have a perimenopausal or menopausal patient with bad migraine headaches – what can you do? Start on 100 mgm 3X/DAY to 5X/DAY
sublingual P4 until symptoms resolve.
(I've just about NEVER seen this fail[62]).

46. WARNING: Average age at menopause in USA? 51 years of age[63] and has an average duration of 4 years (range of 0 to 10 years). And progesterone is the first thing to fall or decline. Usually need progesterone BEFORE this fully gets to you.

47. Progesterone balances estradiol. What? "UNOPPOSED ESTRADIOL (VERY BENEFICIAL WHEN OPPOSED) CAUSES CANCER PROBLEM": Notes on endometrial hyperplasia which is generally considered a precursor to endometrial cancer. The presence of *unopposed estrogen* - which, for example, may result from exogenous estrogen therapy, anovulatory cycles, polycystic ovary syndrome (PCOS), or obesity -- has been shown to increase the likelihood of developing endometrial hyperplasia and cancer[64]. So make sure your patients are on progesterone at healthy optimized levels to prevent this from happening.

48. WARNING: OTC Natural Progesterone Creams (yam or otherwise) usually do NOT work very well, even if patients bathe in the stuff! Why? You cannot come close to getting blood levels up high enough for protection[65] (>10 ng/ml). (Though some of the tiny dose serums are AMAZING!)

49. Hair loss in women (especially older women[66]) can sometimes improve IF you improve their progesterone levels[67].
50. Women with PolyCystic Ovarian Syndrome (PCOS -- a common genetic condition affecting 1 out of 11 women in this country) are all deficient in progesterone and it can competitively lower their supernaturally high testosterone levels (plus improve their insulin sensitivity).
51. Natural progesterone can cause heir regrowth and recovery in women with Androgenetic Alopecia[68] (mainly PCOS women). WARNING: The synthetic MPA in Depo-Provera™ can and does cause hair loss[69] in women while natural progesterone will not or regrows the lost hair[70].
52. Last CRAZY UNEXPECTED BENEFIT: Elevating your progesterone levels assists in the healing and decrease in inflammation of you TMJ pain (Temporomandibular Joint)[71].

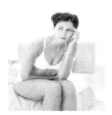

Chapter 4

EASY SUMMARY OF BENEFITS

- Stops or reduces hot flashes
- Stops or reduces night or day sweats
- Reduces risk of breast cancer
- Kills breast cancer cells (causes apoptosis)
- Reduces or reverses fibrocystic breast tissue
- Reduces the risk of heart attacks (reduces coronary artery disease)
- Causes somnolence (sleepiness) and aids in sleep
- Causes weight loss
- Causes increase muscle
- Gets rid of migraines and menstrual headaches in women (not men)
- Shuts down endometriosis
- Halts abnormal uterine bleeding
- Causes hair regrowth (thicker hair)

Chapter 5

SURPRISE BENEFITS

P4 has a number of benefits most patients and physicians find surprising – let's reiterate these. Keeping in mind that levels need to get high enough (varies for different women – everyone's a snowflake remember).

A. IMPROVES LIBIDO

Though a *very* complex issue, when a woman gets her P4 levels back to normal or above (>10ng/mL), then her libido tends to improve[72].

B. RE-MYELINATION OF NERVES

P4 assists in myelination of nerves – so women with low P4 levels often have tingling or burning or a gross neuropathy – and normalizing P4 can reverse this demyelination[73].

C. REDUCES TMJ INFLAMMATION

Lots of studies on PubMed show P4 helps improve temporomandibular joint inflammation[74] (TMJ) and other joint problems.

D. PREVENTS BREAST CANCER

Normalizing P4 levels decreases breast cancer risk[75]. P4 even causes apoptosis (pops) breast cancer cells[76].

E. LOWERS BLOOD PRESSURE

P4 helps lower blood pressure that's high[77] – this is a cool benefit (literally since P4 cools off inflammation in arteries of women).

F. PREVENTS CAD

P4 prevents foam cell formation[78] which lay down plaque in arteries thus preventing coronary artery disease and heart attacks. P4 also lowers cholesterol levels[79], and reduces vascular (endothelial) inflammation[80].

G. PREVENTS STROKE

For the same reasons P4 prevents CAD, P4 prevents strokes, also[81].

H. PREVENTS DVT

P4 not only prevents deep venous thrombosis, but also can reverse clots that are there.

I. CAUSES WEIGHT LOSS

Almost every big study out there P4 causes weight loss[82] and increases muscle development – that's why we often call it a female version of testosterone.

J. PREVENTS MIGRAINES

One of the best benefits of human progesterone is it prevents or even gets rid of migraine headaches in women (not men) – a fact known since 1971[83].

K. PREVENTS OR RELIEVES ENDOMETRIOSIS

There is a current belief among researchers that endometriosis occurs secondary to endometrial resistance to progesterone in some women[84]. The only way known to overcome this resistance is it to take larger doses of progesterone (it's better than narcotics and hysterectomies). Excellent relief often occurs but only with the P4 (bio-equivalent progesterone) not the synthetics.

Chapter 6

WHAT WE TELL PATIENTS

We always advise patients that P4 is not a cure all but can alleviate a lot of symptoms that have tortured them but two things are important:

1. They must take enough to alleviate the symptoms, *and*
2. The compounded progesterone must be of really good quality or they'll pay the price and not get the benefit.

Doses for patients vary (remember that everyone is a snowflake – different levels for different women to get the benefits), so they should not be afraid of taking the progesterone.

Some complain of feeling wobbly or drunk after they take it ad we advise them to take it right before bed, not to drive afterwards, and to go to bed. All seem to comply and love the better sleep they get on P4.

You can get some edema or fluid retention with P4 and no one's quite sure why this happens. We usually give a few Dyazide® (manufactured by GlaxoSmithKline to get rid of this brief edema.

You might also get some nausea, just like when you're pregnant but milder. When your body gets used to this it should get better and go away..

If you take too much P4 you might gain weight so be careful. We advise when starting P4 to eat very carefully – it is a sex hormone, meaning it is anabolic (builds muscle) so in some ways it may increase appetite in order to get more protein into your system. So BE CAREFUL and do not load up on carbohydrates! We tell patients this over and over, reminding them to avoid carbs and to eat protein.

If you have vaginal bleeding that does not stop even with higher doses of P4, then we better look for a fibroid or tumor or polyp – other wise your bleeding should stop completely and periods should be much shorter than typically.

Chapter 7

WAYS TO TAKE P4

SHOTS/INJECTABLE

Used for severe PMS or problems with pregnancy – this is compounded as 100 mg in 1 ml of sterile oil – and you give 1 cc injected intramuscularly (IM) for instant relief.

TOPICAL

Compounded, and made popular by John Lee, MD in the 1990's, this is a widely utilized way to get some progesterone in and to buy it over the counter (OTC). Usually levels don't get very high or even therapeutic (we've not seen it) – this is because you can't absorb enough of the P4 to make a difference *unless* it's very high quality and super micronized – a tricky process at best. The quality of the micronization determines the particle size, this being important because the larger particles (>5 microns) cannot get absorb trough the skin.

Some of the newer topical progesterones we've developed though might be changing this as they give higher blood levels and are very therapeutic.

The topical progesterone does not give a first pass effect through the liver because it does not go through the digestive track.

CAPSULES

Swallow orally. Does give a first pass effect through the liver. Tends to cause weight gain. Again micronization and particle size matter. (You can put lipstick on a pig but it's still a pig, even if it *is* in a capsule!)

TROCHES

"A small medicated lozenge designed to dissolve[85]." Not much different than a triturate, these are just larger. Minimal first pass effect through the liver. Dissolve these under your tongue as best you can – do not swallow while it is in your mouth.

SL TRITURATES

"v. To rub, crush, grind, or pound into fine particles or a powder. n. A triturated substance, especially a powdered drug[86]." Triturate is basically like a troche. Minimal first pass effect through the liver. Dissolve these under your tongue as best you can – do not swallow while it is in your mouth.

WHAT'S AN RDT/ODT?

These are rapid dissolve or oral dissolve triturate designed to dissolve sublingually in just a few seconds – the best way to take progesterone in our opinion.

Dosing of P4 and Vehicle

Usual dose of micronized P4 is 100-200 mg a day (or more, much more) in a triturate or flavored troche. To avoid first pass effect in the liver[87] you dissolve either in your mouth under your tongue (SUBLINGUALLY) until completely dissolved, avoiding drinking or eating anything ten minutes before or after.

Chapter 8

IS THERE A DOWNSIDE TO P4?

There's always a downside to everything, isn't there?

Oral encapsulated progesterone that you swallow can very slightly increase your risk of gallbladder disease or cholecystitis – this is why we tend to use the sublingual triturates.

Factor V Leiden

If you have the genetic disorder called Factor V Leiden, which causes a higher blood pressure and increased risk of clot/stroke/heart attack formation[88] – especially if you give oral estradiol. We'll add oral progesterone to it just to play it safe.

Weight Gain

Too much P4 can cause a need for more protein, which in turn causes a need for increased appetite, which in turn *if you eat too much carbohydrates* then you can get excessive weight gain.

Drowsiness

Directly after taking oral or sublingual progesterone a lot of women get drowsy[89] and want to lie down to go to sleep. This is okay – take it right before bed time. Know that this sleepiness tends to resolve after your body gets used to having higher levels of progesterone in your body.

Wobbly Feeling

Feeling wobbly or intoxicated occur occasionally after higher doses of P4 are taken[90] – DO NOT ATTEMPT TO DRIVE! Be careful and go to bed. This is doesn't happen all the time just enough that new patients call us to ask about it – it goes away after a few months.

Increased Libido

Progesterone (P4) increases libido and desire for women[91]. Sounds fun but can be a problem if you're single or your significant other is not physically or mentally ready for increased "activity." If when you were pregnant, libido improved, then watch out.

Breasts Get Larger and Fluffier

We warn patients about this – progesterone reduces breast density[92] (thus reducing breast cancer risk) and can make them larger and fluffier (lighter). Buy a larger bra usually works. Not to be facetious, just know this can and does occasionally happen.

Chapter 9

HOW IS P4 AVAILABLE?

Progesterone is available a number of different ways – some are a LOT more potent than others – so it's according to your age, your symptoms, your skin condition, and other medical problems.

There are certain times you should *not* take oral progesterone -- when you have a genetic disorder known as Factor V Leiden it's probably not a good idea to take any oral hormones.

PRESCRIPTION VS OTC

Prescription progesterone is either oral (at any concentration) or topical if there's more than 25 mg/gram in a cream or oil – this is a FDA indication though not a ruling, but it's best medico-legally if followed.

We tend to mostly use what are called compounded RDT (rapid dissolve triturate) or ODT (oral dissolve triturate) 200 mg progesterone – and we tell the patient to take them at night. These are for sublingual use and dissolve very quickly and only leave a minimal aftertaste in the mouth. These are used because they enter the blood stream directly and give good levels. These are safe to take up to, and including, the tenth week of pregnancy. These of course are prescription.

Obstetricians like to use compounded progesterone troches for intravaginal application – these are used for maintaining pregnancy but we're not sure why they use these versus the much more palatable sublingual triturate – it seems to be something they learned in residency. We're also unsure why they *then* use synthetics for menopause issues – it's curious and not their compounded vaginal troches. Troches, by the way, can also be used sublingually too though they tend to be awkward but they are flavored and used this way because you can give a bigger dose of progesterone in a troche than in a triturate. These are all prescription medications.

We also rarely use progesterone in oil as an injection though again we see obstetricians doing this quite often. But if a woman is having severe PMS or a migraine 100 mg of P4 on oil (must be compounded) is an option for quick relief. This too is a prescription.

Progesterone is also available in a capsule – either compounded or as Prometrium® manufactured by Solvay Pharmaceuticals. These are prescriptions also and Prometrium®, though very expensive, tends to be covered by insurance. The problem with capsules is that half of the progesterone is eaten up by the liver in what is known as a first pass effect – where substances taken orally must pass through the liver where they are broken down. This is inefficient plus places the unsuspecting women at a very slightly increased risk of gallbladder disease.

If personally compounded, especially at standard concentrations, progesterone in cream at 100 mg/gram of cream is also done by prescription.

Available Over-The-Counter (OTC)

The progesterone in Vitamin E Oil we recently helped design for a prominent essential oils company available without a prescription. Though very potent, it is only at 15 mg/ml of oil to meet FDA requirements but is well worth a try if you cannot get a prescription version.

Also, the progesterone in a cationic gel we've designed for local very prominent skin company is also very potent and they use an electronic device to "push" it into your skin. There are also a number of OTC cream preparations.

Chapter 10

BEST COMPOUNDED VERSIONS OUT THERE?

There are tons of compounding pharmacies out there – remember that before the 1950s all pharmacies were compounding pharmacies. But quality is a huge issue – the quality of the base product that the progesterone is made from, whether soy or yam, and *where* it comes from, is *critical* to the quality.

HOW IT SHOULD BE COMPOUNDED

The compounded progesterone you're being prescribed (or should be prescribed) is a micronized form of natural progesterone. Micronization means the molecules of progesterone must be a certain size for a women to absorb it through her gut lining – we know this is ideally smaller than 5 microns in size. This size of 5 microns is very hard to attain but a few pharmacies are able to do this – they spend a lot of extra effort with what we term "super-micronizing." This means they grind or mill it down further.

The base they use is also critical – yam vs soy – we know of only one pharmacy that uses the soy and they do a very good job but it may not really matter more than the quality of the progesterone. A lot compounding pharmacies are using a cheap Chinese base and we thought that this is a mistake so far. Patients who take compounded P4 based on this base continue to be miserable and call us often complaining of hot flashes and night sweats and migraine headaches. Listen to us pharmacies that are guilty -- WE KNOW WHO YOU ARE AND THIS IS TOTALLY UNACCEPTABLE! Got it?

WHY SOME ARE BETTER?

Because of the care they take in the *further* micronization and in their secret compounding processes they use.

WHAT MAKES SOME THE BEST?

Our two favorite in the USA are:

MedQuest Pharmacy in Bountiful, Utah (http://www.mqrx.com/) – MedQuest is the quiet 800 pound gorilla of the compounding world – everything they make and touch is excellent. When famous actresses talk about progesterone they've been taking, whether they know it or not, they probably are taking MedQuest progesterone. They use an exclusive French soy to make their progesterone and it is *really* good. Try their 200 mg RDT (rapid dissolve tablet) for sublingual use - -it's awesome. Plus they're educational efforts are the best for promoting compounded hormones – they educate both patients and especially physicians. Dr. Purser has educated for MedQuest in the past but has no ownership in this excellent pharmacy. They ship anywhere in the world.

Central Drug in La Habra, California(http://www.anypharmacy.com/) – Central Drug in La Habra has an amazing team of some of the best compounding pharmacists on the planet. Nayan Patel, PhD who runs the pharmacy, originally was schooled at Oxford (as an aeronautical engineer) then decided to use his science background to reshape the compounding world – he and his team are *amazing*. Nayan also teaches about compounding all over the world and is a lecturer at the University of Southern California. When he's not busy teaching he manages to make maybe the best sublingual compounded progesterone on the earth. Made from super-duper-micronized wild yam, Central's P4 dissolves in just a few seconds when it hits the tongue. They call these ODT (oral dissolve tablet) and don't even bother to try to get them under your tongue as they'll be dissolved.

Chapter 11

IS THERE A BIG PHARMA VERSION?

Yes, and we've talked about it throughout this text – Prometrium® manufactured by Solvay Pharmaceuticals (http://www.prometrium.com)– and it's a quality product.

IS IT NATURAL?

We believe it is – it is biologically identical and seems to be made mostly from wild yam.

IS IT EXPENSIVE?

Prometrium® seems to be quite expensive but insurance does tend to cover it. The downside is it only comes in a capsule (in 100 mg and 200 mg doses) and your insurance company will *most likely* limit the number you can take in a day (usually to either one or two at night) – a limitation that most women find annoying because they like to vary their doses according to their symptoms. If this isn't an issue then ask your doctor for Prometrium®.

Chapter 12

Progesterone Practice Gems and Problem Solving

A. Whether capsule, troche, or triturate, give at least 100 mg of human progesterone (P4) every evening.

B. Normal premenopausal progesterone levels (in women) are 4-25 ng/ml. Optimal levels are usually considered to be 10-20 ng/ml.

C. Only get serum progesterone levels not salivary or urinary levels[93] (because they are fairly inaccurate, and indicate a trend more than anything else). This salivary approach, though highly touted on the internet, is not supported in the literature as being accurate. I also spoke at a conference sponsored by MedQuest in 2008 and sat in on a panel where we debated salivary levels (October 3-5, 2008, **New and Functional Approaches To Preventive Medicine** presented in Deer Valley, Utah) – this panel included top physicians in the field of preventive medicine from around the country (including Dr. Purser), Their final conclusion? Salivary levels are still too inaccurate on which to depend.

D. Usually biologically identical human progesterone is given as a flavored triturate or troche under the tongue until it dissolves (no chewing or swallowing if they can help it and do not drink pr eat ten minutes before or after taking).

E. PROBLEM: One of your patients you've started on HRT comes in for her annual exam and on her Pap smear you get *endometrial hyperplasia* – what should you do? Get an intravaginal ultrasound[94] – looking for the endometrial stripe (or a polyp, adenoma, fibroid, cancer), if<5 mm then you're okay – keep treating with HRT with extra progesterone[95]. If >5 mm then stop HRT and refer to an Ob-Gyn.

F. BLEEDING PROBLEM: Your postmenopausal patient has been taking her natural BiEst and Human Progesterone exactly as you prescribed and suddenly she starts bleeding vaginally (a period??!?!) – what do you do? Stop BiEst and double her progesterone (P4) until bleeding stops then go back on BiEst but keep progesterone at double.

> 1. After three months you go back to standard doses of progesterone. Then she starts bleeding vaginally again – what do you do? Stop BiEst and double her progesterone (P4) until bleeding stops then go back on BiEst but keep progesterone at double.

> 2. After three more months you go back to standard doses and she starts bleeding again – what do you do? Get a transvaginal ultrasound[96] to check the endometrial stripe and to rule out polyps, fibroids, adenomas, or endometrial

hyperplasia. If less than 5 mm then start back on BiEst/estradiol and double dose progesterone for 6 months. If stripe is > 5 mm then it might be cancerous[97] so refer to Ob-Gyn as soon as possible.

Short of the referral to an Ob-Gyn another option for fibroids (leiomyomata) is Uterine Artery Embolization (UAE) which is very effective in numerous studies[98]. UAE is where these little polyvinyl alcohol balls are injected into the uterine blood vessels under radiologic guidance (it's a radiology procedure) in order to shrink the fibroids [99].

G. WARNING: ALWAYS GET (from their Ob-Gyn) or PERFORM ANNUAL PAP SMEARS[100] on each patient you have on HRT. Do not refill their prescriptions until you get the result! U.S. Preventive Services Task Force also recommends routine mammography every one to two years for women 40 years and older[101] (no upper limit) – make sure they get this, too.

H. Program 120® Quick Notes on Progesterone:

1. Expect poor absorption (except through mucosal membrane)[102].
2. Dizziness with a high dose[103].
3. Nipple tenderness (rare).
4. Anxiolytic and sedative and hypnotic – good, but if a patient has this effect with their

progesterone then do not use in AM with that patient[104].

5. Oral progesterone undergoes first pass effects in liver – sublingual triturate does not[105].

6. Side effects are usually with oral form only, not SL (sublingual).

7. Men should not use – progesterone severely inflames vascular endothelium[106] and causes impotence!

8. Female postmenopausal patient with insomnia? Change her progesterone to a capsule form and give the 100 mg as Prometrium® orally at night.

I. Hargrove, JT et al from *Infertility and Reproductive Clinics of North America*[107]:

1. Titrate progesterone to pre-menopausal levels. Give 1, 2, 3, or 4 100 mg progesterone a day to achieve this if you need to – don't be shy. Progesterone is protective!

2. Treat menopause as deficiency state.

3. Correct all hormone levels that are deficient (remember: it's the hormonal milieu!).

4. Use human micronized bio-identical hormones[108].

5. Metabolized by normal metabolic pathways.

6. This approach avoids problem causing metabolites.

7. There is absolutely NO reason to not give progesterone to ALL postmenopausal women – hysterectomy or not.

8. There is no good reason NOT to give these bio-identical estrogens and progesterone every day[109]. *Do not cycle – give them all every day.*

J. PREGNANCY PROBLEM: You have a patient on HRT and her level of progesterone comes back >100 ng/ml, why? She's pregnant until proven otherwise.

K. PMS PROBLEM: You have a pre-menopausal patient with bad PMS symptoms, what can you do? Use P4 in a 100 mg compounded vaginal suppository for 7-14 days (prior and up to menstruation).

L. POST-PARTUM BLUES PROBLEM: You have a patient with bad post-partum depression, what can you do? Start on 100 mg TID sublingual P4 for 7 days, then BID SL P4 for 7 days, then QD SL P4 for 7 days.

M. HOT FLASHES PROBLEM: You have a perimenopausal patient with bad hot flashes (Inhibin A in decline from the ovary is *now* felt to cause hot flashes), night sweats, and vaginal dryness -- what can you do? Start on 100 mg TID sublingual P4 for 7 days (or until symptoms resolve) realizing they won't cycle (but who cares? Right?).

N. MIGRAINE PROBLEM: You have a perimenopausal or menopausal patient with bad migraine headaches -- what can you do? Start on 200 mg RDT TID to 5X DAY sublingual P4 until symptoms resolve.

O. Average age at menopause in USA? 51 years of age[110] and has an average duration of 4 years (range of 0 to 10 years).

P. UNOPPOSED CAUSES CANCER PROBLEM: Notes on endometrial hyperplasia which is generally considered a precursor to endometrial cancer. The presence of *unopposed estrogen* - which, for example, may result from exogenous estrogen therapy, anovulatory cycles, polycystic ovary syndrome (PCOS), or obesity -- has been shown to increase the likelihood of developing endometrial hyperplasia and cancer[111]. So make sure your patients are on progesterone at healthy optimized levels to prevent this from happening!

Q. The Pap test is not that helpful in identifying women who have endometrial hyperplasia -- who are at increased risk for endometrial neoplasia. In one study, the presence of normal endometrial cells in postmenopausal women not on hormonal therapy was associated with a 19 percent risk for endometrial hyperplasia or carcinoma[112].

R. OTC Natural Progesterone Creams (yam or otherwise) older models do NOT work, even if patients bathe in the stuff! Why? Older creams can give only minimal relief, unless you supply a lot you cannot come close to getting blood levels up even minimally. The newer oil based or gel based progesterones we've recently helped design and tested get much higher levels than some oral forms – this is due to the extensive extra micronization we put the progesterone through before we finalize the production. Try these first, especially if you cannot get your doctor to prescribe oral versions that meet your requirements.

S. NO LIBIDO DUE TO YASMIN® PROBLEM: Final note: Yasmin® is currently the Program 120® team favorite birth control pill because of its very positive anti-androgenic effects (drosperinone and ethinyl esradiol). But remember those anti-androgenic effects will potentially dry up libido[113].

T. Though P4 reduces the risk of strokes and heart attacks and DVTs, we always give aspirin (when possible) and lots of fish oil because if they ever get a clot they might try to blame it on the P4 – this is just added insurance against this ever happening.

Chapter 13

PATIENT EXAMPLES

Note that for any of these patients topical progesterone is okay.

A. 14 year old female with severe PMS

   Her mom or dad should give her a small dose (50 mg?) of sublingual when she becomes emotionally unbearable or has bad cramps or stomach aches – usually these girls will go lay down, take a brief nap, then wake up very happy. It's kinda weird.

B. 23 year old female with migraines

   She probably has PMS also and heavy crazy periods – she could take a 100 or 200 mg sublingual progesterone RDT when she has a headache but ideally she should probably take this every day so she never ever has another migraine. We are not sure why this progesterone trick and treatment has been so squelched because it's so easy to rid women of migraines with P4.

C. 45 year old female with hot flashes and night sweats after a hysterectomy.

She should also take lots of 200 mg RDTs – until she is symptom free. Make sure she's also on estradiol orally if possible (see our **Program 120** textbook for more info)..

D. 19 year old with hot flashes, night sweats and no periods

TROUBLE! She needs an ultrasound and careful evaluation as to why her ovaries have shut down. Sounds like a primary (genetic or ovarian trauma?) or secondary (pituitary?) ovarian failure or insufficiency and you better figure out which. This girl will need some help and probably has a lot of other symptoms so start digging.

E. 64 year old female with hot flashes and history of fibromyalgia

Women with fibro receive so much benefit from P4 – they should all be on it. These women are miserable souls and need all the help they can get.

F. 62 year old with no hot flashes or night sweats – went through easy menopause

These are the hardest to treat. What do you do? They still need the hormones as they still have prevention issues but it's often difficult to convince them of this fact.

G. 52 year old with history of progesterone receptor positive breast cancer

These women will also benefit from progesterone RDT and should have lots of it. With the receptors in place the progesterone will cause apoptosis of these cancer cells and act as a chemo agent.

This is an Interactive Book with FREEBIES!

For your free downloadable PDF on Dr. Purser's Labs and how to get them through his affiliate lab site, please visit our website and sign up for his email newsletter (then the Lab PDF is downloadable for FREE!).

Just scan this code with your smart phone QR Reader:

Or go to (it's SUPER EASY):

http://www.drpurser.com

TERMINOLOGY

BID – Take two times a day

DVT- deep venous thrombosis

mg – milligram

MPA—medroxyprogesterone acetate – synthetic progestational agent

ODT – oral dissolve triturate

OTC – over the counter – does not require a prescription

P4 – biologically identical progesterone – also called bio-identical progesterone – identical to what a female human's ovaries elute.

RDT – rapid dissolve triturate

TID – take three times a day

INDEX

References

[1] Hargrove, JT; Osteen, KC. An Alternative Method of Hormone Replacement Therpay Using the Natural Sex Steroids. Infertility and Reproductive Medicine Clinics of North America. Volume 6, Number 4, October 1995.

[2] [No authors listed] Medroxyprogesterone acetate. IARC Monogr Eval Carcinog Risk Chem Hum. 1979 Dec;21:417-29.

[3] Klaiber EL; Vogel W; Rako S. A critique of the Women's Health Initiative hormone therapy study. Fertil Steril. 2005; 84(6):1589-601 (ISSN: 1556-5653).

[4] Thomas T, Rhodin J, Clark L, Garces A. Progestins initiate adverse events of menopausal estrogen therapy. Climacteric. 2003 Dec;6(4):293-301.

[5] Campagnoli C, Clavel-Chapelon F, Kaaks R, Peris C, Berrino F. Progestins and progesterone in hormone replacement therapy and the risk of breast cancer. J Steroid Biochem Mol Biol. 2005 Jul;96(2):95-108.

[6] Cushman M, Legault C, Barrett-Connor E, et al. Effect of postmenopausal hormones on inflammation-sensitive proteins: the Postmenopausal Estrogen/Progestin Interventions (PEPI) Study. Circulation. 1999;100:717-722.

[7] Clark MK, Sowers M, Levy B, Nichols S. Bone mineral density loss and recovery during 48 months in first-time users of depot medroxyprogesterone acetate. Fertil Steril. 2006 Nov;86(5):1466-74.

[8] Archer B, Irwin D, Jensen K, Johnson ME, Rorie J. Depot medroxyprogesterone. Management of side-effects commonly associated with its contraceptive use. J Nurse Midwifery. 1997 Mar-Apr;42(2):104-11.

[9] Klaiber EL; Vogel W; Rako S. A critique of the Women's Health Initiative hormone therapy study. Fertil Steril. 2005; 84(6):1589-601 (ISSN: 1556-5653).

[10] Online at www.nlm.nih.gov/medlineplus/ency/article/003714.htm. Accessed 2006 Oct 12.

[11] Campagnoli C, Clavel-Chapelon F, Kaaks R, Peris C, Berrino F. Progestins and progesterone in hormone replacement therapy and the risk of breast cancer. J Steroid Biochem Mol Biol. 2005 Jul;96(2):95-108.

[12] Attia MA, Zayed I. Thirteen-weeks subcutaneous treatment with high dose of natural sex hormones in rats with special reference to their effect on the pituitary-gonadal axis. II. Progesterone. Dtsch Tierarztl Wochenschr. 1989 Oct;96(9):445-9.

[13] Effects of estrogen or estrogen/progestin regimens on heart disease risk factors in postmenopausal women. Writing Group for the PEPI Trial. JAMA. 1995;273:1389-96.

[14] Hargrove JT, Maxson WS, Wentz AC, Burnett LS. Menopausal hormone replacement therapy with continuous daily oral micronized estradiol and progesterone. Obstet Gynecol. 1989 Apr;73(4):606-12.

[15] Sitruk-Ware R, Bricaire C, DeLignieres B, et al. Oral Micronized progesterone. Bioavailability pharmacokinetics, pharmacological and therapeutic implications—A Review, Contraception. 1987; 36:373-402.

[16] WEN-SEN LEE, CHAO-WEI LIU, SHU-HUI JUAN, YU-CHIH LIANG, PEI-YIN HO, AND YI-HSUAN LEE. Molecular Mechanism of Progesterone-Induced Antiproliferation in Rat Aortic Smooth Muscle Cells. Endocrinology 144(7):2785–2790. Copyright © 2003 by The Endocrine Society doi: 10.1210/en.2003-0045.

[17] McCrohon JA; Nakhla S; Jessup W; Stanley KK; Celermajer DS. Estrogen and progesterone reduce lipid accumulation in human monocyte-derived macrophages: a sex-specific effect. Circulation. 1999; 100(23):2319-25 (ISSN: 0009-7322).

[18] Campagnoli C, Clavel-Chapelon F, aaks R, Peris C, Berrino F. Progestins and progesterone in hormone replacement therapy and the risk of breast cancer. J Steroid Biochem Mol Biol. 2005 Jul;96(2):95-108.

[19] Cowan LD, Gordis L, et al. Breast cancer incidence in women with a history of progesterone deficiency. Am J Epidemiol. 1981 Aug;114(2):209-17. Cowan LD, Gordis L, et al. Breast cancer incidence in women with a history of progesterone deficiency. Am J

Epidemiol. 1981 Aug;114(2):209-17.

[20] Cowan LD, Gordis L, et al. Breast cancer incidence in women with a history of progesterone deficiency. Am J Epidemiol. 1981 Aug;114(2):209-17.

[21] Friel AM, Zhang L, et al. Progesterone receptor membrane component 1 deficiency attenuates growth while promoting chemosensitivity of human endometrial xenograft tumors. Cancer Lett. 2014 Oct 7. pii: S0304-3835(14)00577-1. doi: 10.1016/j.canlet.2014.09.036.

[22] Murkes D, Lalitkumar PG, et al. Percutaneous estradiol/oral micronized progesterone has less-adverse effects and different gene regulations than oral conjugated equine estrogens/medroxyprogesterone acetate in the breasts of healthy women in vivo. Gynecol Endocrinol. 2012 Oct;28 Suppl 2:12-5.

[23] Lydeking-Olsen E, Beck-Jensen JE, Setchell KD, Holm-Jensen T. Soymilk or progesterone for prevention of bone loss--a 2 year randomized, placebo-controlled trial. Eur J Nutr. 2004 Aug;43(4):246-57.

[24] Randall TC, Kurman RJ. Progestin treatment of atypical hyperplasia and well-differentiated carcinoma of the endometrium in women under age 40. Obstet Gynecol 1997;90:434-40.

[25] Fraser IS. Regulating menstrual bleeding. A prime function of progesterone. J Reprod Med 1999;44(2 suppl):158-64.

[26] Arafat ES, Hargrove JT, Maxson WS, Desiderio DM, Wentz AC, Andersen RN. Sedative and hypnotic effects of oral administration of micronized progesterone may be mediated through its metabolites. Am J Obstet Gynecol. 1988 Nov;159(5):1203-9.

[27] Vanselow W, Dennerstein L, Greenwood KM, de Lignieres B. Effect of progesterone and its 5 alpha and 5 beta metabolites on symptoms of premenstrual syndrome according to route of administration. J Psychosom Obstet Gynaecol. 1996 Mar;17(1):29-38.

[28] Maxson WS. The use of progesterone in the treatment of PMS. Clin Obstet Gynecol. 1987:30:465-477

[29] Ahlgrimm, M. (May 2003). Managing pms and perimenopause symptoms The role of compounded medications, Advance for Nurse Practitioners, (11)5, p. 53.

[30] Hitchcock CL, Prior JC. Oral micronized progesterone for

vasomotor symptoms--a placebo-controlled randomized trial in healthy postmenopausal women. Menopause. 2012 Aug;19(8):886-93. doi: 10.1097/gme.0b013e318247f07a.

[31] Goddard LM1, Ton AN, et al. Selective suppression of endothelial cytokine production by progesterone receptor. Vascul Pharmacol. 2013 Jul-Aug;59(1-2):36-43. doi: 10.1016/j.vph.2013.06.001.

[32] APGAR, B.S., GREENBERG, G. Practical Therapeutics Using Progestins in Clinical Practice. AFP - October 15, 2000.

[33] Fitzpatrick, LA; Pace, C; Wiita, B. Comparison of Regimens Containing Oral Micronized Progesterone or Medroxyprogesterone Acetate on Quality of Life in Postmenopausal Women: A Cross-Sectional Survey. Journal of Women's Health & Gender-Based Medicine. May 2000, Vol. 9, No. 4 :381 -387.

[34] Davis SR, Guay AT, Shifren JL, Mazer NA. Endocrine aspects of female sexual dysfunction. J Sex Med. 2004 Jul;1(1):82-6.

[35] Hargrove JT, Maxson WS, Wentz AC, Burnett LS. Menopausal hormone replacement therapy with continuous daily oral micronized estradiol and progesterone. Obstet Gynecol. 1989:73: 606-612.

[36] Spark MJ Mpharm, Dunn RA Bpharm Hons, et al. Women's Perspective on Progesterone: A Qualitative Study Conducted in Australia. Int J Pharm Compd. 2009 July-Aug;13(4):345-349.

[37] Miller BE, De Souza MJ, et al. Sublingual administration of micronized estradiol and progesterone, with and without micronized testosterone: effect on biochemical markers of bone metabolism and bone mineral density. Menopause. 2000 Sep-Oct;7(5):318-26.

[38] Clayton AH. The pathophysiology of hypoactive sexual desire disorder in women. Int J Gynaecol Obstet. 2010 Jul;110(1):7-11. doi: 10.1016/j.ijgo.2010.02.014.

[39] Prior JC. Progesterone for Symptomatic Perimenopause Treatment - Progesterone politics, physiology and potential for perimenopause. Facts Views Vis Obgyn. 2011;3(2):109-20.

[40] Prior JC. Progesterone for Symptomatic Perimenopause Treatment - Progesterone politics, physiology and potential for perimenopause. Facts Views Vis Obgyn. 2011;3(2):109-20.

[41] Zumpe D, Clancy AN, Michael RP. Progesterone decreases mating and estradiol uptake in preoptic areas of male monkeys. Physiol Behav. 2001 Nov-Dec;74(4-5):603-12.

[42] O'Leary P, Feddema P, Chan K, Taranto M, Smith M, Evans S. Salivary, but not serum or urinary levels of progesterone are elevated after topical application of progesterone cream to pre-and postmenopausal women. Clin Endocrinol (Oxf). 2000 Nov;53(5):615-20.

[43] Ruiz AD, Daniels KR. The effectiveness of sublingual and topical compounded bioidentical hormone replacement therapy in postmenopausal women: an observational cohort study. Int J Pharm Compd. 2014 Jan-Feb;18(1):70-7.

[44] Ruiz AD, Daniels KR. The effectiveness of sublingual and topical compounded bioidentical hormone replacement therapy in postmenopausal women: an observational cohort study. Int J Pharm Compd. 2014 Jan-Feb;18(1):70-7.

[45] Wren BG, Day RO, McLachlan AJ, Williams KM. Pharmacokinetics of estradiol, progesterone, testosterone and dehydroepiandrosterone after transbuccal administration to postmenopausal women. Climacteric. 2003 Jun;6(2):104-11.

[46] Warren MP, Shantha S. Uses of progesterone in clinical practice. Int J Fertil Womens Med. 1999 Mar-Apr;44(2):96-103.

[47] Bitran, D.; Shiekh, M.; McLeod, M. Anxiolytic Effect of Progesterone is Mediated by the Neurosteroid Allopregnanolone at Brain GABAA Receptors. Journal of Neuroendocrinology, Volume 7 Page 171 - March 1995 doi:10.1111/j.1365-2826.1995.tb00744.x, Volume 7, Issue 3.

[48] Simon JA. Micronized progesterone: vaginal and oral uses. Clin Obstet Gynecol 1995;38:902-14.

[49] Zitzmann M; Erren M; Kamischke A; Simoni M; Nieschlag E. Endogenous progesterone and the exogenous progestin norethisterone enanthate are associated with a proinflammatory profile in healthy men. J Clin Endocrinol Metab. 2005; 90(12):6603-8 (ISSN: 0021-972X).

[50] Schumacher M, Mattern C, et al.. Revisiting the roles of progesterone and allopregnanolone in the nervous system: resurgence of the progesterone receptors. Prog Neurobiol. 2014 Feb;113:6-39. doi: 10.1016/j.pneurobio.2013.09.004.

[51] Melcangi RC, Giatti S, et al. Levels and actions of progesterone and its metabolites in the nervous system during physiological and pathological conditions. Prog Neurobiol. 2014 Feb;113:56-69. doi:

10.1016/j.pneurobio.2013.07.006.

[52] Melcangi RC, Giatti S, et al. Levels and actions of progesterone and its metabolites in the nervous system during physiological and pathological conditions. Prog Neurobiol. 2014 Feb;113:56-69. doi: 10.1016/j.pneurobio.2013.07.006.

[53] Schumacher M, Mattern C, et al. Revisiting the roles of progesterone and allopregnanolone in the nervous system: resurgence of the progesterone receptors. Prog Neurobiol. 2014 Feb;113:6-39. doi: 10.1016/j.pneurobio.2013.09.004.

[54] El-Etr M, Rame M, et al. Progesterone and nestorone promote myelin regeneration in chronic demyelinating lesions of corpus callosum and cerebral cortex. Glia. 2015 Jan;63(1):104-17. doi: 10.1002/glia.22736.

[55] Mitro N, Cermenati G, et al. Neuroactive steroid treatment modulates myelin lipid profile in diabetic peripheral neuropathy. J Steroid Biochem Mol Biol. 2014 Sep;143:115-21. doi: 10.1016/j.jsbmb.2014.02.015.

[56] Peterson TC, Hoane MR, et al. A COMBINATION THERAPY OF NICOTINAMIDE AND PROGESTERONE IMPROVES FUNCTIONAL RECOVERY FOLLOWING TRAUMATIC BRAIN INJURY. J Neurotrauma. 2014 Oct 14.

[57] Hargrove, J, Osteen, K. An alternative method of hormone replacement therapy using the natural sex steroids. *Infertility and Reproductive Medicine Clinics of North America* 1995;4:653-74.

[58] Hargrove JT, Maxson WS, Wentz AC, Burnett LS. Menopausal hormone replacement therapy with continuous daily oral micronized estradiol and progesterone. Obstet Gynecol. 1989 Apr;73(4):606-12.

[59] Hargrove JT, Maxson WS, Wentz AC, Burnett LS. Menopausal hormone replacement therapy with continuous daily oral micronized estradiol and progesterone. Obstet Gynecol. 1989 Apr;73(4):606-12.

[60] Al-Sabbagh M1, Lam EW, Brosens JJ. Mechanisms of endometrial progesterone resistance. Mol Cell Endocrinol. 2012 Jul 25;358(2):208-15. doi: 10.1016/j.mce.2011.10.035.

[61] Valenzuela SK. The power of natural progesterone: treating hormone-related postpartum depression. Midwifery Today Int Midwife. 2012 Autumn;(103):22-5.

[62] Borsook D, Erpelding N, et al. Sex and the migraine brain. Neurobiol Dis. 2014 Aug;68:200-14. doi:

10.1016/j.nbd.2014.03.008.

[63] Rubin, R. Out of the hot flash and into the fire. USA TODAY. [online] Available at www.usatoday.com/news/health/2005-03-29-menopause_x.htm.

[64] Chudnoff, SG. Ask the Experts about Gynecology and Reproductive Endocrinology. From Medscape Ob/Gyn & Women's Health. Endometrial Hyperplasia. [online] Available at www.medscape.com/viewarticle/507187. Accessed 2006 Oct 12.

[65] O'Leary P, Feddema P, Chan K, Taranto M, Smith M, Evans S. Salivary, but not serum or urinary levels of progesterone are elevated after topical application of progesterone cream to pre-and postmenopausal women. Clin Endocrinol (Oxf). 2000 Nov;53(5):615-20.

[66] Jamin C. [Androgenetic alopecia]. [Article in French] Ann Dermatol Venereol. 2002 May;129(5 Pt 2):801-3.

[67] Diamanti-Kandarakis E, Tolis G, Duleba AJ. Androgens and therapeutic aspects of antiandrogens in women. J Soc Gynecol Investig. 1995 Jul-Aug;2(4):577-92.

[68] Jamin C. [Androgenetic alopecia]. [Article in French] Ann Dermatol Venereol. 2002 May;129(5 Pt 2):801-3.

[69] Archer B, Irwin D, et al. Depot medroxyprogesterone. Management of side-effects commonly associated with its contraceptive use. J Nurse Midwifery. 1997 Mar-Apr;42(2):104-11.

[70] Diamanti-Kandarakis E, Tolis G, Duleba AJ. Androgens and therapeutic aspects of antiandrogens in women. J Soc Gynecol Investig. 1995 Jul-Aug;2(4):577-92.

[71] Madani AS, Shamsian AA, et al. A cross-sectional study of the relationship between serum sexual hormone levels and internal derangement of temporomandibular joint. J Oral Rehabil. 2013 Aug;40(8):569-73. doi: 10.1111/joor.12074.

[72] Stuckey BG. Female sexual function and dysfunction in the reproductive years: the influence of endogenous and exogenous sex hormones. J Sex Med. 2008 Oct;5(10):2282-90.

[73] De Nicola AF, Labombarda F, et al. Progesterone neuroprotection in traumatic CNS injury and motoneuron degeneration. Front Neuroendocrinol. 2009 Jul;30(2):173-87.

[74] Kramer PR, Bellinger LL. The effects of cycling levels of 17beta-estradiol and progesterone on the magnitude of temporomandibular

joint-induced nociception. Endocrinology. 2009 Aug;150(8):3680-9.
[75] Online at www.nlm.nih.gov/medlineplus/ency/article/003714.htm. Accessed 2006 Oct 12.
[76] Arruvito L, Giulianelli S, Flores AC, Paladino N, Barboza M, Lanari C, Fainboim L. NK cells expressing a progesterone receptor are susceptible to progesterone-induced apoptosis. J Immunol. 2008 Apr 15;180(8):5746-53.
[77] Langrish JP, Mills NL, et al. Cardiovascular effects of physiological and standard sex steroid replacement regimens in premature ovarian failure. Hypertension. 2009 May;53(5):805-11.
[78] WEN-SEN LEE, CHAO-WEI LIU, SHU-HUI JUAN, YU-CHIH LIANG, PEI-YIN HO, AND YI-HSUAN LEE. Molecular Mechanism of Progesterone-Induced Antiproliferation in Rat Aortic Smooth Muscle Cells. Endocrinology 144(7):2785–2790. Copyright © 2003 by The Endocrine Society doi: 10.1210/en.2003-0045.
[79] McCrohon JA, Nakhla S, et al. Estrogen and progesterone reduce lipid accumulation in human monocyte-derived macrophages: a sex-specific effect. Circulation. 1999 Dec 7;100(23):2319-25.
[80] Wassmann S, Nickenig G. Pathophysiological regulation of the AT1-receptor and implications for vascular disease. J Hypertens Suppl. 2006 Mar;24(1):S15-21.
[81] McCrohon JA, Nakhla S, et al. Estrogen and progesterone reduce lipid accumulation in human monocyte-derived macrophages: a sex-specific effect. Circulation. 1999 Dec 7;100(23):2319-25.
[82] Chmouliovsky L, Habicht F, James RW, Lehmann T, Campana A, Golay A. Beneficial effect of hormone replacement therapy on weight loss in obese menopausal women. Maturitas. 1999 Aug 16;32(3):147-53.
[83] Somerville BW. The role of progesterone in menstrual migraine. Neurology. 1971 Aug;21(8):853-9.
[84] Young SL, Lessey BA. Progesterone function in human endometrium: clinical perspectives. Semin Reprod Med. 2010 Jan;28(1):5-16.
[85] No Author listed. Definition of Troche. [online] Available at http://www.medterms.com/script/main/art.asp?articlekey=19526. Accessed 2010 April 09.
[86] No Author listed. Definition of Triturate. [online] Available at http://medical-dictionary.thefreedictionary.com/triturate. Accessed

2010 April 09.

[87] Simon JA. Micronized progesterone: vaginal and oral uses. Clin Obstet Gynecol 1995;38:902-14.

[88] Kujovich JL. Prothrombin Thrombophilia.In: Pagon RA, Bird TC, Dolan CR, Stephens K, editors. GeneReviews [Internet]. Seattle (WA): University of Washington, Seattle; 1993-. Accessed 2010 Apr 25.

[89] Arafat ES, Hargrove JT, Maxson WS, Desiderio DM, Wentz AC, Andersen RN. Sedative and hypnotic effects of oral administration of micronized progesterone may be mediated through its metabolites. Am J Obstet Gynecol. 1988 Nov;159(5):1203-9.

[90] Mitre EI, Figueira AS, Rocha AB, Alves SM. Audiometric and vestibular evaluation in women using the hormonal contraceptive method. Braz J Otorhinolaryngol. 2006 May-Jun;72(3):350-4.

[91] Stuckey BG. Female sexual function and dysfunction in the reproductive years: the influence of endogenous and exogenous sex hormones. J Sex Med. 2008 Oct;5(10):2282-90.

[92] Santos SJ, Aupperlee MD, et al. Progesterone receptor A-regulated gene expression in mammary organoid cultures. J Steroid Biochem Mol Biol. 2009 Jul;115(3-5):161-72.

[93] O'Leary P, Feddema P, Chan K, Taranto M, Smith M, Evans S. Salivary, but not serum or urinary levels of progesterone are elevated after topical application of progesterone cream to pre-and postmenopausal women. Clin Endocrinol (Oxf). 2000 Nov;53(5):615-20.

[94] Berek JS, Hacker NF, eds. Practical gynecologic oncology. 2d ed. Baltimore: Williams & Wilkins, 1994:285-326, with information from Karlsson B, Granberg S, Wikland M, Ylostalto P, Torvid K, Marsal K, et al. Transvaginal ultrasonography of the endometrium in women with postmenopausal bleeding: a Nordic multicenter study. Am J Obstet Gynecol 1995;172:1488-94.

[95] Chudnoff, SG. Ask the Experts about Gynecology and Reproductive Endocrinology. From Medscape Ob/Gyn & Women's Health. Endometrial Hyperplasia. [online] Available at www.medscape.com/viewarticle/507187. Accessed 2006 Oct 12.

[96] Berek JS, Hacker NF, eds. Practical gynecologic oncology. 2d ed. Baltimore: Williams & Wilkins, 1994:285-326, with information from Karlsson B, Granberg S, Wikland M, Ylostalto P, Torvid K,

Marsal K, et al. Transvaginal ultrasonography of the endometrium in women with postmenopausal bleeding: a Nordic multicenter study. Am J Obstet Gynecol 1995;172:1488-94.

[97] Goldstein SR, Zeltser I, Horan CK, Snyder JR, Schwartz LB. Ultrasonography-based triage for perimenopausal patients with abnormal uterine bleeding. Am J Obstet Gynecol 1997; 177: 102-8.

[98] Wachter, K. UAE Shows Some Advantage Over Myomectomy. Family Practie News, Volume 35, Issue 5, Page 59 (01 March 2005).

[99] Walker WJ, McDowell SJ. Pregnancy After Uterine Artery Embolization for Leiomyomata: a Series of 56 Completed Pregnancies. Am J Obstet Gynecol. 2006;195:1266-1271.

[100] [no authors listed] U.S. Preventive Services Task Force. Screening for Cervical Cancer. Release Date: January 2003. Available online at www.ahrq.gov/clinic/uspstf/uspscerv.htm. Accessed 2006 Oct 12.

[101] [no authors listed] U.S. Preventive Services Task Force. Screening for Breast Cancer. Release Date: February 2002. Available online at www.ahrq.gov/clinic/uspstf/uspsbrca.htm. Accessed 2006 Oct 12.

[102] Wren BG, Day RO, McLachlan AJ, Williams KM. Pharmacokinetics of estradiol, progesterone, testosterone and dehydroepiandrosterone after transbuccal administration to postmenopausal women. Climacteric. 2003 Jun;6(2):104-11.

[103] Warren MP, Shantha S. Uses of progesterone in clinical practice. Int J Fertil Womens Med. 1999 Mar-Apr;44(2):96-103.

[104] Bitran, D.; Shiekh, M.; McLeod, M. Anxiolytic Effect of Progesterone is Mediated by the Neurosteroid Allopregnanolone at Brain GABAA Receptors. Journal of Neuroendocrinology, Volume 7 Page 171 - March 1995 doi:10.1111/j.1365-2826.1995.tb00744.x, Volume 7, Issue 3.

[105] Simon JA. Micronized progesterone: vaginal and oral uses. Clin Obstet Gynecol 1995;38:902-14.

[106] Zitzmann M; Erren M; Kamischke A; Simoni M; Nieschlag E. Endogenous progesterone and the exogenous progestin norethisterone enanthate are associated with a proinflammatory profile in healthy men. J Clin Endocrinol Metab. 2005; 90(12):6603-8 (ISSN: 0021-972X).

[107] Hargrove, J, Osteen, K. An alternative method of hormone replacement therapy using the natural sex steroids. *Infertility and Reproductive Medicine Clinics of North America* 1995;4:653-74.

[108] Hargrove JT, Maxson WS, Wentz AC, Burnett LS. Menopausal hormone replacement therapy with continuous daily oral micronized estradiol and progesterone. Obstet Gynecol. 1989 Apr;73(4):606-12.

[109] Hargrove JT, Maxson WS, Wentz AC, Burnett LS. Menopausal hormone replacement therapy with continuous daily oral micronized estradiol and progesterone. Obstet Gynecol. 1989 Apr;73(4):606-12.

[110] Rubin, R. Out of the hot flash and into the fire. USA TODAY. [online] Available at www.usatoday.com/news/health/2005-03-29-menopause_x.htm.

[111] Chudnoff, SG. Ask the Experts about Gynecology and Reproductive Endocrinology. From Medscape Ob/Gyn & Women's Health. Endometrial Hyperplasia. [online] Available at www.medscape.com/viewarticle/507187. Accessed 2006 Oct 12.

[112] Ng AB, Reagan JW, Hawliczek S, Wentz BW. Significance of endometrial cells in the detection of endometrial carcinoma and its precursors. Acta Cytol 1974;18:356-61.

[113] Schneider HP. Androgens and antiandrogens. Ann N Y Acad Sci. 2003 Nov;997:292-306.

Made in the USA
Lexington, KY
25 March 2019